Brain Bursts For All

A new concept, simple or profound

EILEEN FRY

CP
THE CHOIR PR

First published in the United Kingdom in 2023 by

The Choir Press

ISBN 978-1-78963-380-1

Introduction

This book is to provide you with fun, pleasure and your own *Brain Burst*. It is for the creative mind. Study each story along with the illustration as a separate entity, pause for a while, then grab a pen.

If you are leading a group into creative writing or thought processing, it is up to you to go on a journey.

The group could be schoolchildren, or seniors needing guidance, or just on their own they could study it and find pleasure.

The book could be a useful gift to a loved one then you can share your own *Brain Bursts* together. If it makes you smile, then it is worthwhile.

Finally, I must remind you that however you use the book, the conclusions you reach are subject to your own interpretation.

Enjoy!

Love and blessings

Eileen Fry

Eileen Fry is an established author, but this book is a new concept. Her previous books have all been historical ghost stories and childhood autobiographies. She worked for many years with children with special needs and then most recently cared for her husband with Alzheimer's.

Dedication

This book is dedicated to Mike, my husband.

For ten years, he carried the weight of Alzheimer's. This time was still an important part of his life. It was still a time to smile, though the strangest thing of all is the changes in lifestyle. They become unbelievable. Most of all, a dependence on others' love and kindness has many different manifestations. I know there were happy moments for Mike, and we cling to those memories as an important part of his life story.

Brain

This little book is a glimpse of small brain bursts, which happen when we open the door to our imagination. Just by gazing at a random picture, we can open up many unknown paths. Memories we had previously tucked away. You too can relax and enjoy the pleasure of this experience. Look at a picture for a while then pick up a pen. What an adventure! Please try.

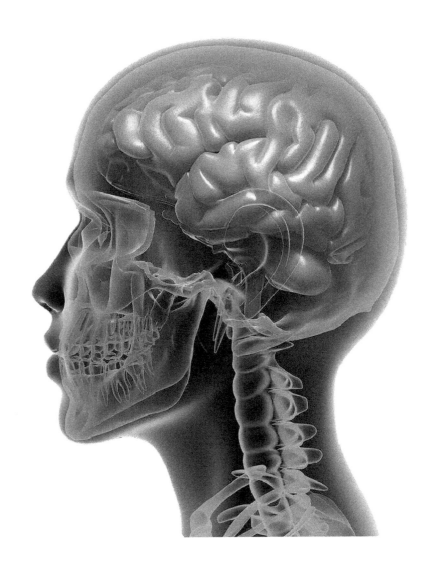

A Robin

A perky passing robin decided to pause, perch and sing. To Ben the gardener, Robin was a regular friend, ever waiting for a worm.

Robin, to Grace, was a mouth to feed. It gave her pleasure to see him peck on the scattered crumbs she provided.

Robin, to Gordon, was a reminder of past times spent with Betty, when they travelled to the forest armed with binoculars and a keen curiosity.

Robin, to Julia, meant the day ahead would be a lucky one full of sunshine.

Robin, to Mary, signified past schooldays. A timid nun confided in her that his red breast represented the blood of Christ on the cross.

Robin makes a lot of people happy. He also gives his name to football and rugby teams. Up the Robins! How versatile is that?

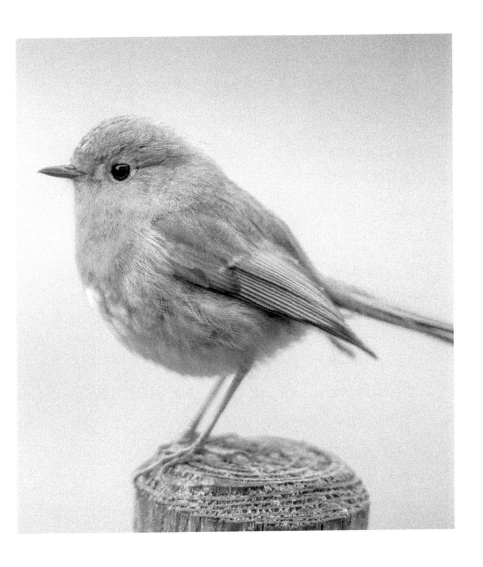

The Woodcarver

He sits amid the chippings, quietly
whittling wood.

Making shapes, gently carving patterns
hard and good.

Why does he find it easy when others find it
hard?

I could never use wood, so it's not written
on my card.

We all have a gift, so they say, even when
it's hard to find.

Somehow, it's fitted into that space we
sometimes call our mind.

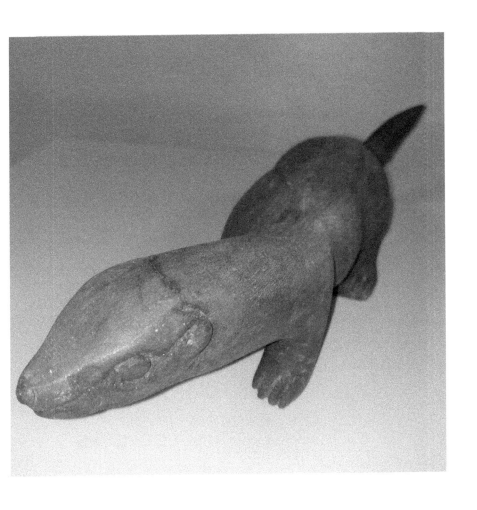

A Dog Named Harry

Just a little dog named Harry. A small, perky, white, furry companion. He gazed up at owner Pat. His bright quizzical eyes said it all. What adventure shall we have today? His head was cocked on one side. It was obvious he needed an immediate answer. Do we go now or later? Will you please grab my new red lead! I am ready. My feet need to run run run. To explore new paths and feel the wind.

"Sorry, Harry. Mummy is not too well today. I feel a bit giddy, I am out of sorts. My legs are wobbly, bones are creaky. Old age is getting in the way. I would love to chase up the hill with you, share a bracing walk, meet friends along the way, just as we did when you were a pup. Today, I must rest, and instead show you the garden, with its old familiar pebbles and plants. You may even be able to chase a squirrel. Perhaps tomorrow will be better."

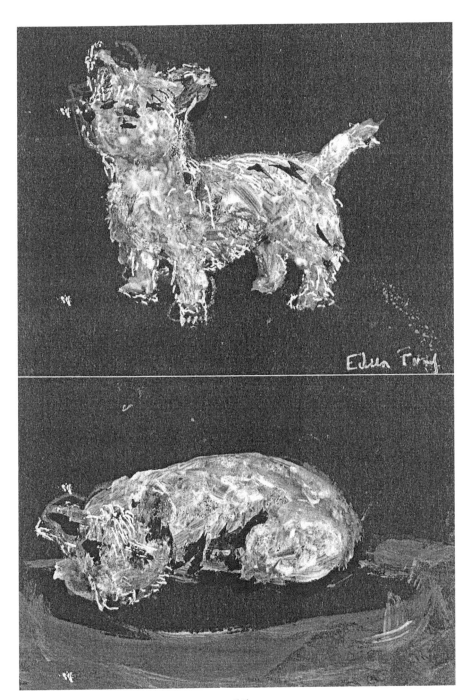

Edna Ford

11

The Sound of Silence

The music stopped; chattering ceased. Doors slammed shut; my ears pricked up. Then I heard it. The Sound of Silence.

At first, I was fearful and felt alone. Where and what was this new place? Sitting quietly, I closed my eyes. No longer fearful, the peace absorbed me.

The sun was shining high on the hill. Nothing moved or stirred in my new place.

Time meant nothing at all. My imaginative heart was restored.

Joy, bliss and peace were now my home. The pleasure was mine for the asking.

I promised myself I would return again.

If only I could find the time!

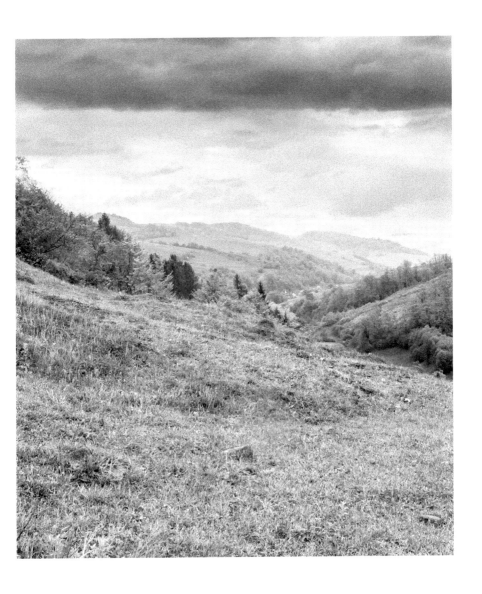

13

Slowly Going Under

A balmy summer evening sitting outside
The Red Lion at Wainlode with a drink.

This was, however, no ordinary Saturday
night. This was after the Big Flood of 2007.
This was when Nature decided we were in
for a surprise! Roads became rivers.
Tewkesbury was drowning; lives were in
peril; sirens wailed. Homes were lost or
ruined.

Heroes were made as if fuelled by
adrenalin and, motivated by love. They put
their own lives at risk to save others.

We heard later that at two in the morning
- loud bangs, groans, as if in its death
throes - the brave little boat finally gave up
the fight. It was gone, never to be seen
again. That's all I know. It remains gone
forever. It was no great ship of merit. Not
the Titanic. Just a small boat lost and gone
forever, but I still remember that night and
my special photo.

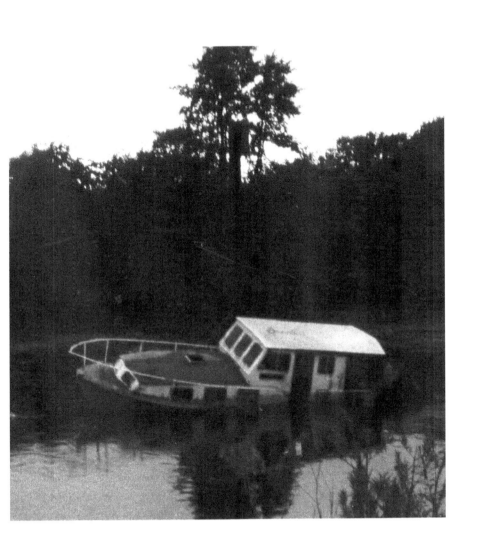

What is Time?

Time is a second

Seconds make a minute

Minutes soon become an hour

Hours turn into days

Days counted in seven become a week.

Four weeks are then a month

Months transform to years

Years become a lifetime

Treasure each second before it speeds the
journey of your lifetime.

TIME

Time is a second

Time is a lifetime

Time is precious, to be used wisely.

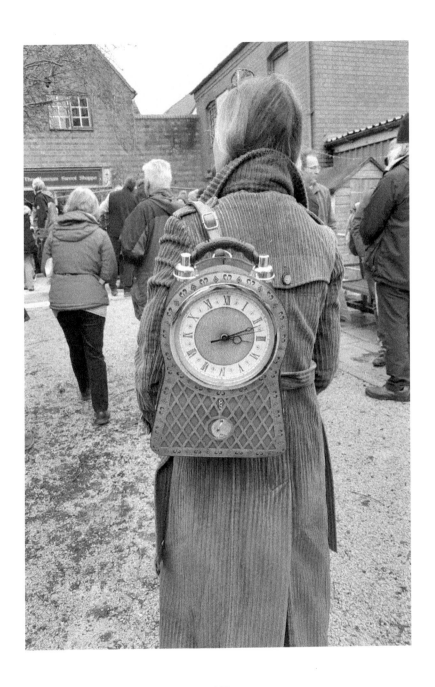

Piano Power

The black polished piece of furniture stands
grandly in the corner.

Looking good but alone, silent, ignored.

The maestro approaches, music in hand.

He takes his place on the stool.

Lifting the lid, revealing a smiling set of keys.

Quickly, the room becomes alive.

An eager audience now awaits.

Music at last, emotions aroused.

Now the singing becomes spontaneous.

Some are even swaying to the rhythm.

Songs and words become alive.

Music and souls become as one.

Audience participation unstoppable.

Eventually, the sounds cease.

The maestro is played out.

My soul is transformed; my heart has a new
beat.

This is the power of music.

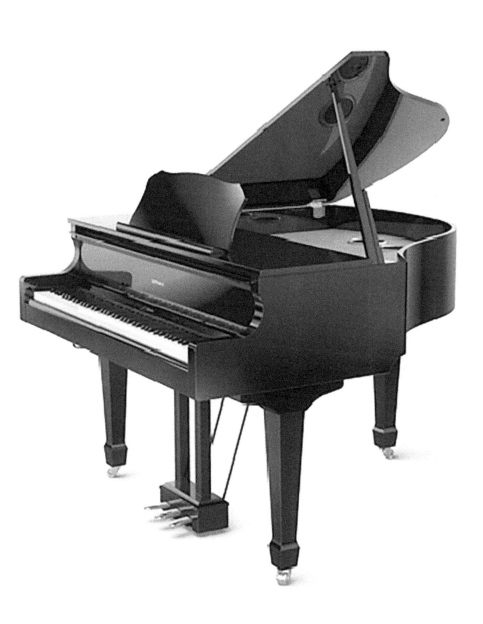

The Value of a Newspaper

Once, a newspaper was cherished, read and then passed around. Politics in faraway London; local happenings; births, deaths, marriages and adverts. What to buy and where. A schoolboy with a big sack on his back. Sleepy eyes found the route. The sound of the letterbox became an early-morning call. Sunshine or hail, the paper must be there.

Now comes further enlightenment. Press for info, instant knowledge. See it happen anyhow, anywhere.

Did it happen or is it false news?

More confused, more facts, less wisdom.

Better to use the paper once again to wrap up fish and chips or light the fire.

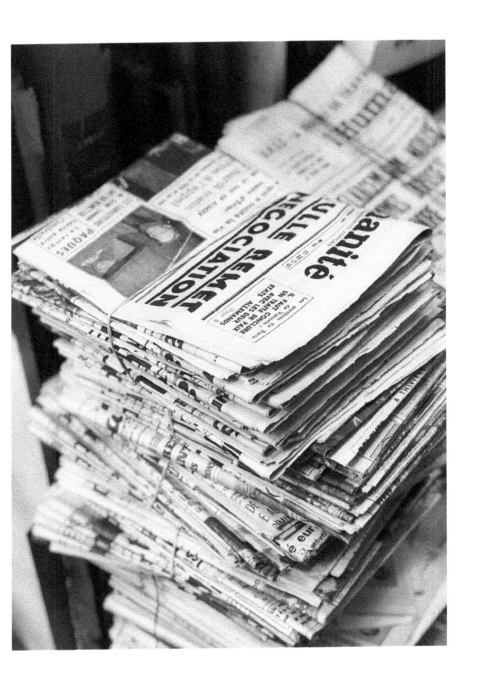

Dazzled by the Sun

My very first seaside holiday beckoned.
Eagerly, we set off in the Morris Minor car.
Waiting for the very first crossing of the
day. Ryde on the Isle of Wight was the
destination. This needed a trip across the
sea. Wow! Eventually, we settled in our
Puckpool chalet. This was in a wonderful
holiday camp.

Cases unpacked, we were eager to see the
beach. Beach was a place yet to be
discovered. I was mesmerised by the scene.
So vast the water, so blue and gold. The sun
was hot as we were covered with its
warming rays. This was truly amazing. I
stood stock-still and felt its comforting
embrace, such a golden new experience.
This sun could not be surpassed. In a flash,
it came to me. This was exactly the same
sun I had left behind at home. Now it was
with me still.

How could that be?

What an amazing world!

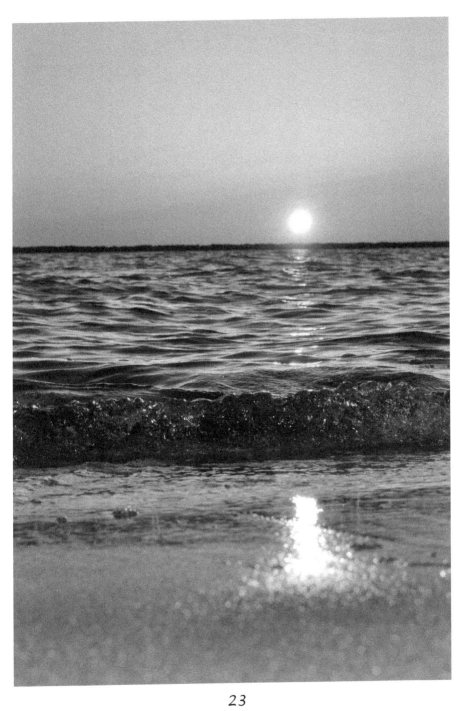

Darren's Taxi

The new car stood on the drive.
Perfect shiny new for all to see.
Papers now signed, cash transferred.
The test drive was perfect.
Steering good to the touch. Excellent!
The owner was happy and proud.
As the car sped along, so did the years.
Careful maintenance and regular checks.
The attention meant it was still in good
running order.

What of the owner and his condition?
How was his bag of bones getting along?
Through neglect of maintenance, he was
not firing on all cylinders.
Our bodies need regular check-ups.
Warning signs acknowledged, and dealt
with.
Leaks and spillages must be controlled.
Our body is our temple.
You are more valuable than a car.
You are unique and irreplaceable.
Keep on taking the tablets!

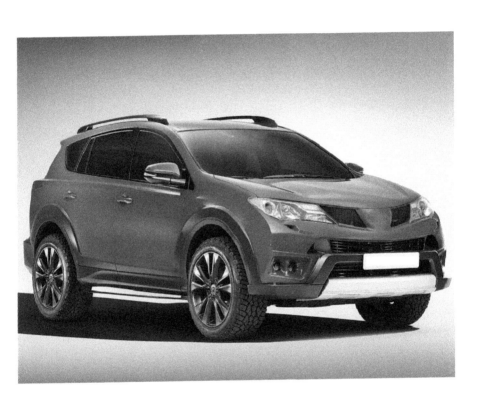

The Golf Ball, 1944

I begged my mum and dad to take me to Mitcham Common. I needed to run with grass under my feet.

I rushed to the golf course beyond.

Two men were swinging clubs.

It looked an impossible task.

The distance was long and the hole so small.

Sometimes, it did happen. Two grown men shouting for joy in a war-torn time.

Now, however, I rooted around in the bush.

I had discovered a small lonely golf ball.

It must have been hiding there some time, perhaps frightened by the sounds of war.

I took the ball home in my pocket. It was beginning to rot with age. I stripped it right down to its core. A myriad of rubber bands revealed.

I had discovered the heart of golf.

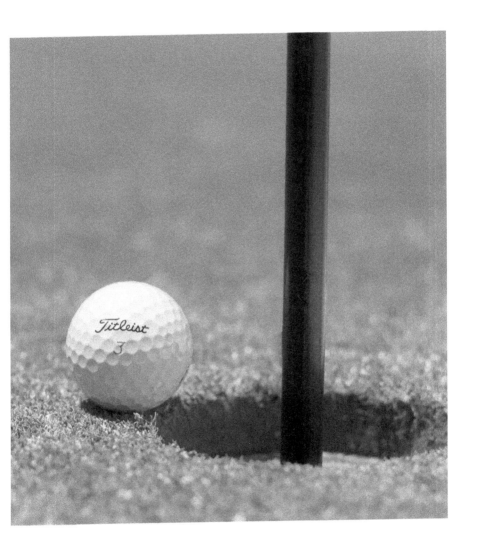

The Glass

The glass was used for drinking; it saw many a merry lip. Happy laughter filled the room as the tippler took a sip. Now it stands silent on a shelf. Antique is now its name, longing to serve a purpose, not a silent empty fame.

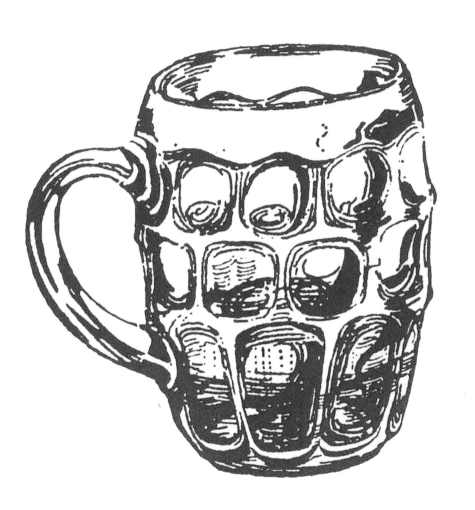

The Globe

A bright shiny globe upon a stand; we know now the earth is round. Many years ago, others saw our world as flat, before the truth was found. They would argue with assertion and claim the truth their right. No one would believe otherwise; it was not in their sight. Just how many other things are there for us now to discover? Who knows, but one day we may find out how to love each other.

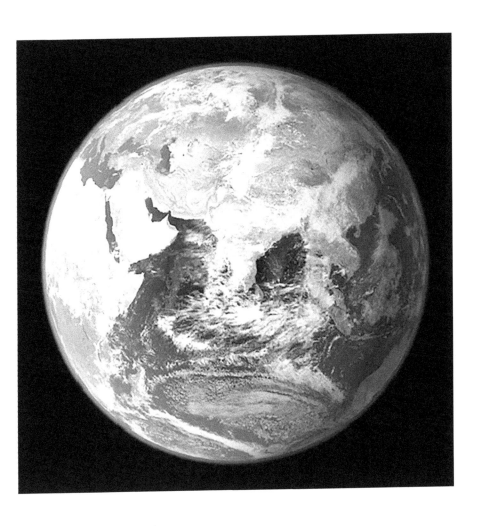

Mitzi

Mitzi was really only half a dog. The other half was more than human. She knew her purpose in life. Her job was to stay ever close to Vyv. To watch and protect her. It was her raison d'être.

She sat on the wheelchair as Vyv took her for a daily ride. Mitzi never moved, just looked around, her little body firmly fixed. She ignored dogs completely and only glanced at other humans. There will never be another Mitzi.

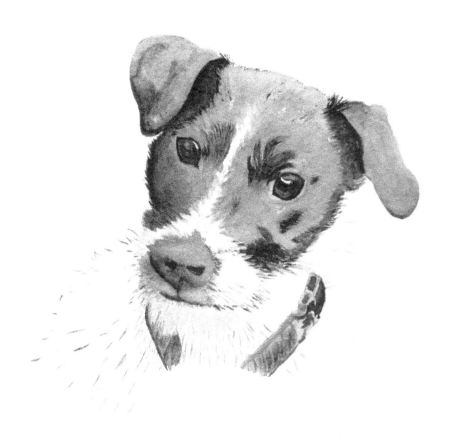

The Year of the Rabbit

It was early evening inside a house in Stoke-on-Trent.

Three hungry kids home from school were waiting to be fed. Dad David heard a strange noise in the garden.

He opened the door to the dark, frosty outside. Something moved. A large black rabbit was about to strike lucky.

David and wife Louise brought in the intruder together, and decided to give Rabbit a new home. In spite of the disapproval of two resident self-opinionated cats.

By chance, their first pet pre-children had been a large WHITE rabbit.

In faraway CHINA on 22nd January 2023, they celebrated the Year of the Rabbit and the year of HOPE.

The same HOPE mentioned in a book belonging to David.

Any place, anywhere.

We need HOPE.

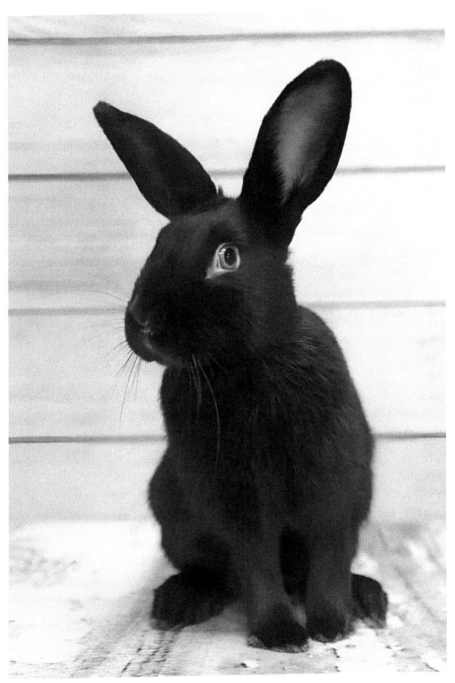

Dick Whittington

Just a boy setting off to be an apprentice in London. Leaving behind his life on the farm and the rolling hills of Gloucestershire. Was it ever in his plan to become a friend to a king and a mayor of London? Did he ever dream of being the main player in the pantomime? I don't think so. He was just a lad needing the companionship of his cat. We shall never know.

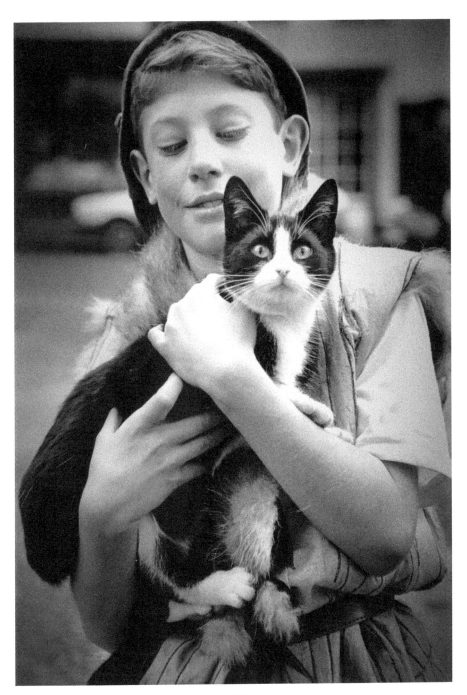

Sam in the Lighthouse

The lighthouse came into view.

It appeared to be black and white in the troubled night sky. The sea rolled, frothy, angry, and in control, but ...

Now we knew at last we were going home.

The bright flashing beams sent a message of blessed assurance.

We passed around the keg and raised our voices in praise. We thanked God for the old sailor, who now spends lonely days in a lighthouse just to see us safely home. Soon we would be on dry land, but he would still be lighthouse bound.

Three cheers for Sam.

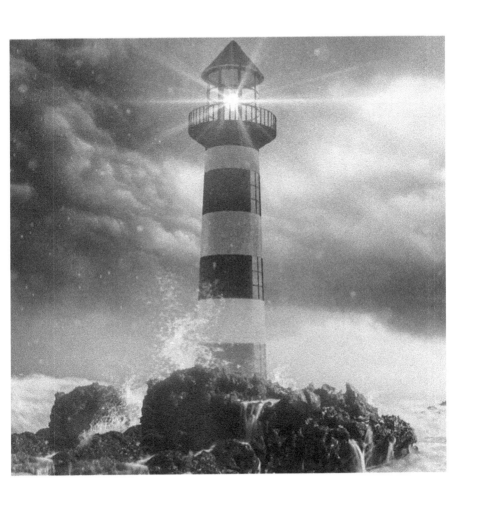

An Unexpected Wassail

Phillip made his way down a Saturday-afternoon shopping street. He stopped in awe as before his unprepared eyes, a white-bearded elderly man, playing a frantic flute, danced before him. Dressed in a long white smock and large hat, he was really frolicking. A lady in equally rustic dress danced with him. Following, with gust melodies, was quite a similar crowd.

For a moment, Phillip feared for his sanity. Then he too was invited to follow the throng. Throwing caution to the wind, he agreed. The joyous line re-entered the old house came out into ? rear garden. The singing continued at the same time as a large jug of cider was passed along. As if giving a perfectly logical explanation, it was revealed that the group were blessing the apple tree. They were singing the Wassail Song. All this took place on a January afternoon in old Gloucester.

Ah, that's all right then, thought Phillip.

Just another day.

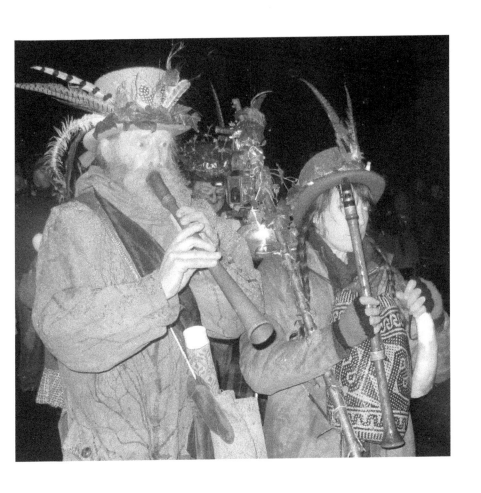

Samantha's Snowdrops

Two days before Christmas and at 5.30 a.m., Sam set off on her regular morning jog, needing to feel fresh and set her mind free before confronting the busy day ahead. She embraced the silence with gentle steps. The path grew clearer in the frosty mist. Suddenly Sam stopped in her tracks. Her Slavonic pale blue eyes grew wide as they spotted an unexpected delight. Next to the track, growing proudly and serenely, stood a generous clump of beautiful snowdrops. They commanded attention. Sam rested her long legs and reached for her phone. Excitedly, she recorded her surprise encounter with Mother Nature.

Later on that day, at 4 p.m., a great man slipped away. Sam had formed a close connection to him and helped him on his journey. She felt later the snowdrops had given her a silent message.

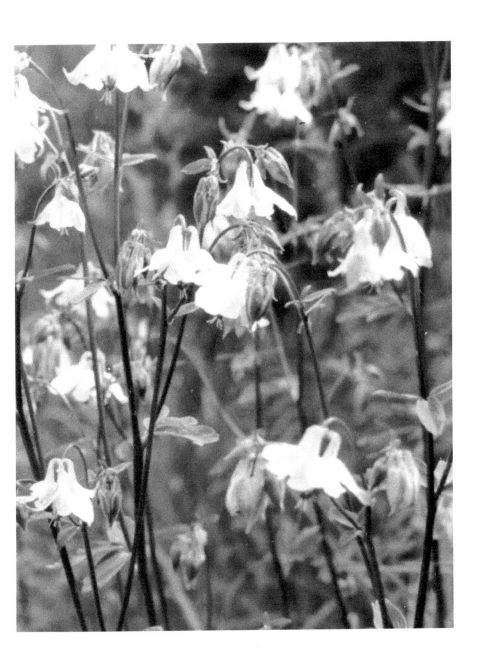

43

Old Friends

Old friends are wonderful; they make a base for what we become. Sometimes, however, when you least expect it, you meet up with a stranger and make an instant connection. This stranger can influence your future and help you re-evaluate your past. Life can be an exciting adventure. I met my latest new friends following a trip to the aisles at Tesco.

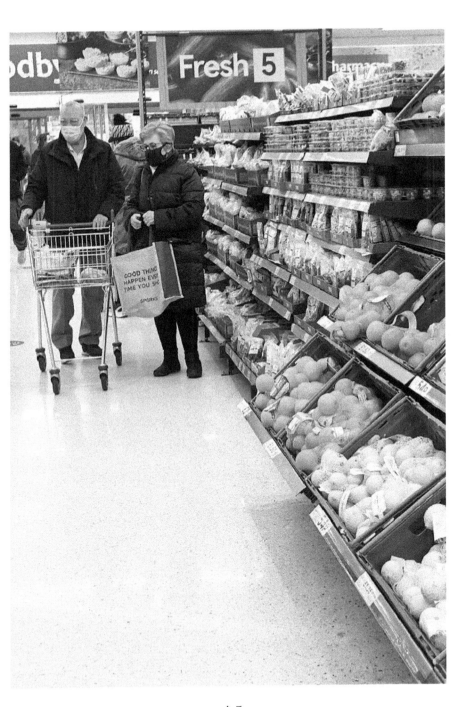

My COVID Colour

It was surreal. Too many questions. What is COVID? How do we cope? Answers came from all directions. Medical advice leaflets, posters. The media was on fire with info. How to deal with doom, gloom and disaster. But what about me? Decisions were endless. The answer came in a flash. Before I succumb to whatever, I need to make a statement. I will dye my hair.

With my mask firmly in place, I entered Tesco. A young girl stood before me. She chose a red colour with a smile on her face. So I did it. I too bought the same shade. In one day, I transformed from white to effervescent pink. No going back.

Anticipating instant incarceration or at least derision, I stepped out into my new world. No longer was I an ancient white blob. I was transformed into a mild talking point. Now I was at least acknowledged, if only with mild amusement.

I felt liberated. Yippee!

It was my COVID colour.

Bring it on!

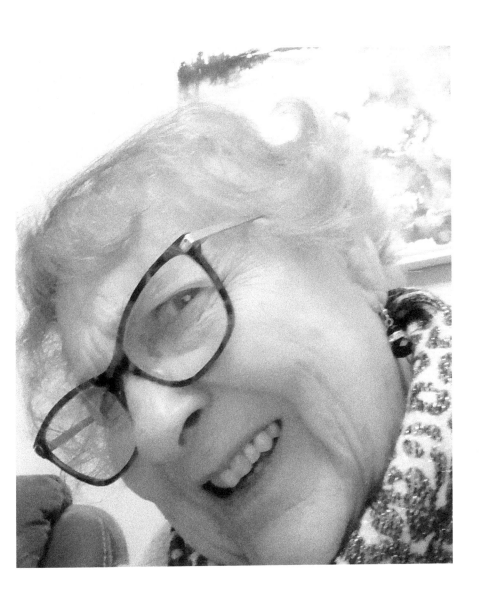

The Spirit of Christmas

With a friendly smile, the young mother told a stranger, 'My son says he likes the colour of your hair.' Stopping at once, barriers down, the conversation became animated.

The result was surprising. Days later, the mother was escorting the lady to Gloucester Cathedral. Her son was a young chorister singing at Evensong. At 5 p.m., the service began. The two women glanced at each other in a timeless heavenly rapture.

*

Two weeks passed. It was Christmas Day. The old lady sat with the family around the table laden with a Christmas meal 'par excellence'. Young and old chatted enthusiastically. It was a picture of traditional fun. The conversation was endless.

The young chorister's random remark had resulted in a kindness to a stranger.

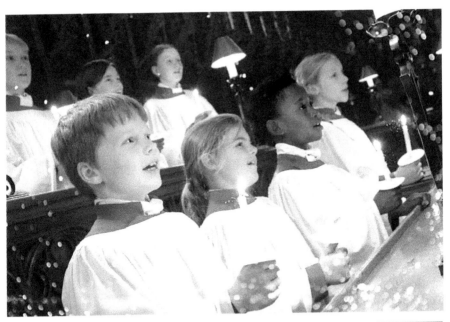

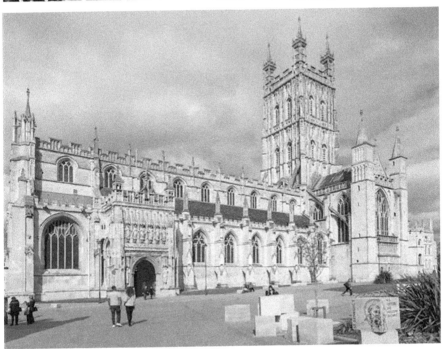

You're Only Old Once

You're only old once so make the most of complaining about the weather. It's too cold, too hot or windy.

Say how you creak as you get up from the chair. Why not?

Tell the children how hard it was in the past. No money, no food, socks needed darning, queues for most things, etc., etc.

No one had tablets like they do now, taking the darn things everywhere. Now you need them to keep you going, or even on the run.

You're only old once, so give it a go, to say thank you and please, ?s we were taught long ago.

Tell someone you love them and value them too. Sing all the old songs as long as you can, even if it's croaky.

Dance with your stick. Cheat at a quiz. Dye your hair. Wear purple. Go to a pantomime. You're only old once.

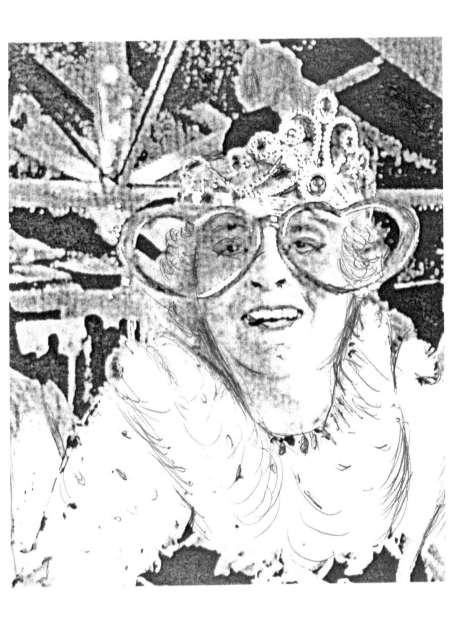

Clouds

To see a cloud formation is a joy.

The farmer gazes up to foretell the weather.

Dark clouds mean rain.

Light fluffy clouds rising high, what bliss!
Warmth and fresh air.

Now Man in his debatable wisdom has
created a new cloud.

This will store data we may never use or
need again.

Gallons of water will be needed for how
long?

Can Man compete with a natural creation?

I think not!

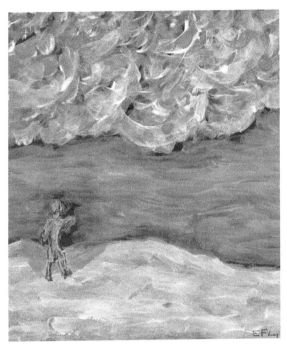

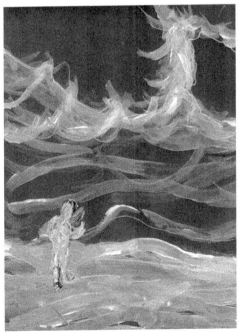

53

Think Before You Wrap

Casually, I was packing a Christmas gift for my artist friend Rosemary. We have shared many life experiences, big and small. Whatever the situation, it always leads to long in-depth discussions. Casually, I tossed in a fir cone. It had been around my apartment many years, resting wherever it fell, a pretty reminder of one of nature's ornaments. I even wrapped it in paper whilst admiring its pretty bottom, as one does.

*

Christmas over, Rosemary thanked me for the gift and shared with me the tale of a man from Pisa named Fibonacci. In the Middle Ages, he studied plants and patterns in nature, including snails. This mathematical pattern is in all nature's creation, leading to a common creator known to some as GOD.

Well, I am pleased she enjoyed the gift. So think before you wrap.

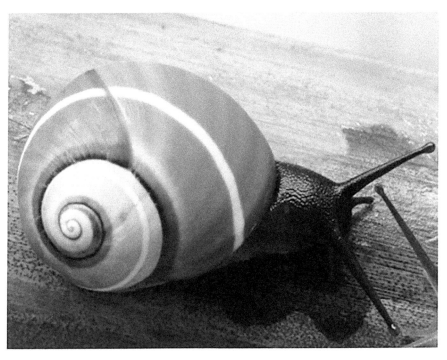

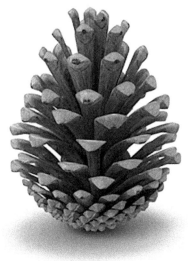

Was There a Plan?

Two more young immigrants trudged along the road. Jo had to return to his place of birth to sign papers, for the government; otherwise, he would have no status. They had not been married long and the young girl was heavily pregnant. Where would the baby be born? The authorities did not really care.

Transport was a problem; they had no money for that. The real name of the father of the baby had been a question. Now the marriage was legal so Jo's name was on the form.

The social worker overlooking the registration felt a justified concern for the future child. Outsiders muttered how it was an irresponsible act to bring a baby into such a troubled world. No money, no home, no job prospects and certainly no stable government. How would this new baby find any place in such a struggling world?

On the form they wrote down the name of the new bride. It was Mary.

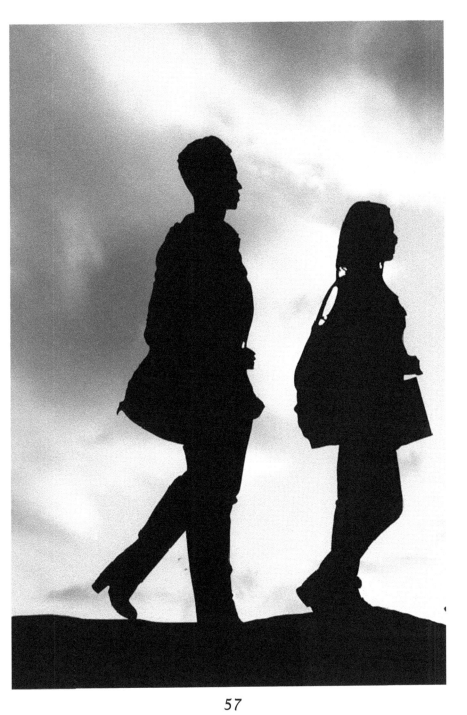

A Policy Shift

Testing,

Underground testing.

What reactions nuclear weapons?

Race with arms.

What options?

Multipolar world

Drastic solutions.

Nuclear weapons for all.

Earth rebels

Nature mutilated,

God rages.

World destroyed.

What was man?

Just a memory returned to dust.

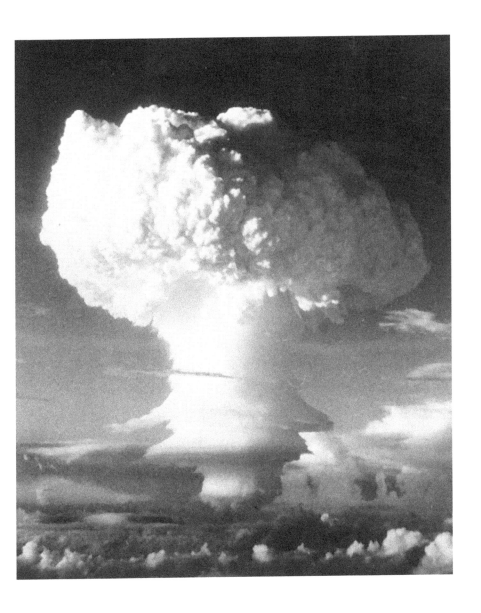

The Silent Witness

I was a newly planted sapling, eager to grow and strengthen. The young couple came close to me as they cuddled and made plans.

*

Years passed. The same couple in the same place could be heard shouting in anger. Silently, I gave out my peace. They were calm again. Now they bring along their grandchildren for a picnic and to reminisce. I am still here to give them my peace and protection.

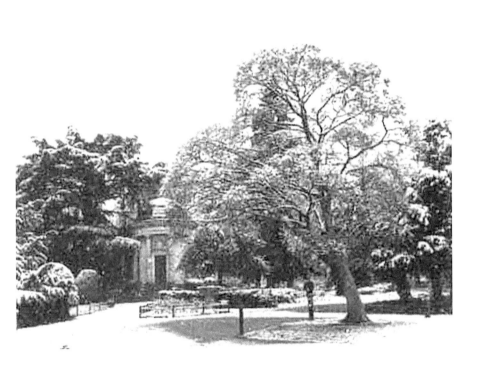

Snow

A winter scene of snow. To one happy child, it meant fun building a snowman. The best ever! He returned home to a new pair of slippers and a warm drink. Amazing.

To the refugee, it meant another hungry, cold and desperate day.

To the little bemused bird, it meant searching harder for tasty worms.

Fun or famine,

Nature presents us with our own choices.

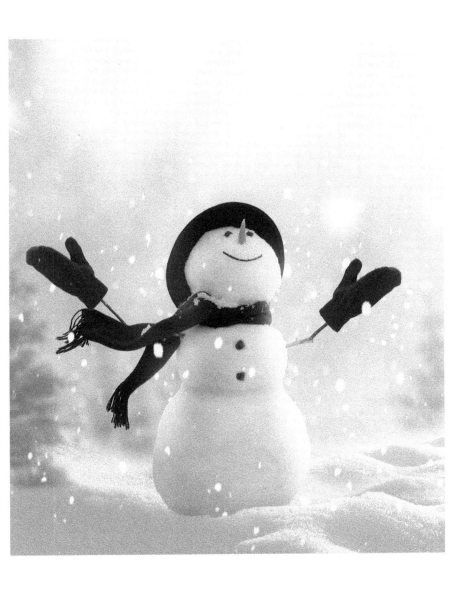

The Lost Lottery Ticket

No response - not from the media.

No response - from messages or social media.

A forgotten lottery ticket. Now declared a winner, a million-pounds temptation, just lost, but where?

Who knows?

Who cares?

Has a life been ruined by the loss?

Has a life been saved from making the wrong decision?

Does the purchaser know?

Does the purchaser even care?

We shall never know.

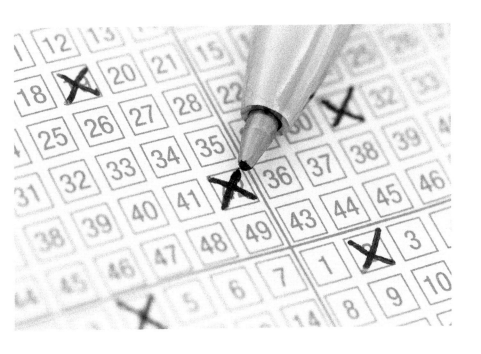

The Open Door

A sign reads, 'Everyone Welcome'.

'Everyone but me,' she scoffed.

'Things' got worse, muddled, confusion. No answer; she still passed by. Drowning in a sea of despair. On impulse, she passed through the door, crossed the line. One small step brought her back.

Just look for a door.

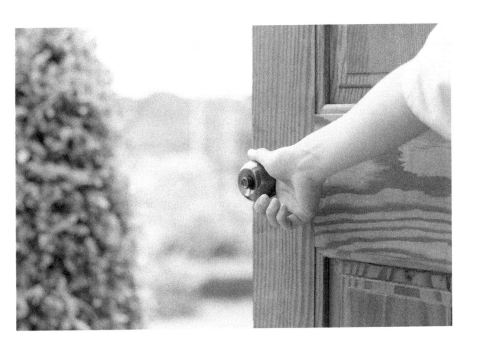

The Ladder of Success

Years ago, Frederick decided he wanted to be a success in life. His ambition was to climb the ladder of success; he would be a leader of men. He would fight for power and rights.

He joined the military; the uniform was impressive. His men followed his commands.

Deciding to overcome the enemy, Frederick led the men into battle. He was invincible.

Fearless Frederick climbed the ladder of confrontation.

Frederick died!

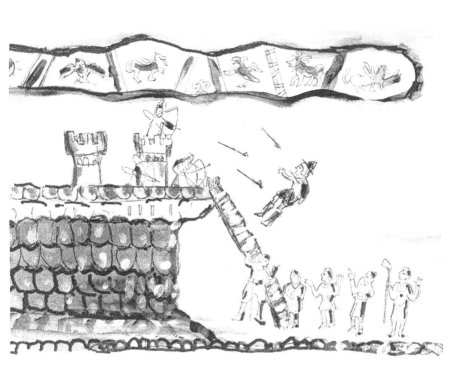

The Blackbird

The night was dark, but a blackbird sang.

Surprised but inspired, a young man from Liverpool penned a song.

A song which gave enjoyment and pleasure to many.

Sometime later, still holding that song in her memory, an artist took out her brush, then painted the blackbird.

The music was still with her.

Paul's song, the Blackbird and Rosemary became connected in spirit again.

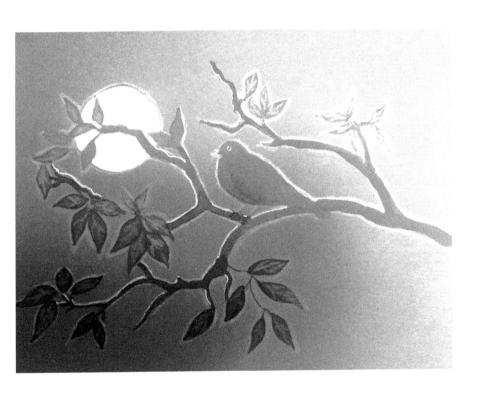

Remembrance Sunday

It was a bit cloudy as we set off. My son of sixty-one years deigned to take me for a car ride. As we left the houses of Swindon behind and made our way through Wroughton, then rose higher and higher along the narrow country lane, the sun began to break through the puffy clouds. The car was brought to a stop at the top of Barbary Castle.

Sitting there in our comfort zone, we began to chat about old times. Somehow, a rare opportunity for mother and son. As we gazed at the view from our very high point, the sun appeared and every cloud disappeared. It was a warm sunny day, the sort of day you dream about as you plan any trip into the countryside but rarely experience in perfection, but this was certainly the best day ever weather-wise, even though it belied the November date on the calendar. I really felt this was a day like no other. One that would forever be in my thoughts as if it had lasted a whole month. Time was surely losing any meaning. After all, time is perhaps only a concept.

In the middle of the field in front of us there were two kites flying, strangely enough flown by two middle-aged men who were unconnected in any way. The man on the left was successfully flying his kite. It gracefully dipped and circled in an effortless, gentle way at a good height. We then noticed that the attached strings were supporting seven beautiful remembrance poppies, the red colour reflecting the sun's rays in a very special way. This was a day I will treasure forever.

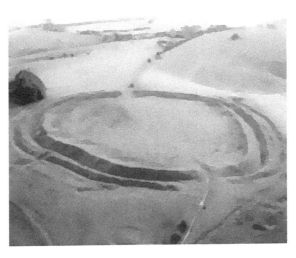

Matts poem

If you come to Scotland you'd better beware
Of a terrifying creature one millimetre
square

Highland midges are not dangerous things
But given a chance they are irritation on
wings

When the wind drops they rise
To swarm in front of your eyes

And its hard to show grace
When they start eating your face

So if you can't run and hide
And prefer being outside

The best thing to do with a dastardly
midge
Is give it a slap and make it go squidge.

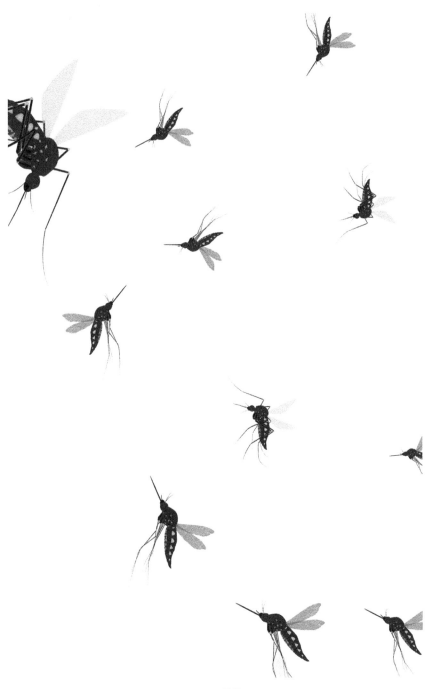

What King Charles III did

It was May 2023 in England, we paused for a party. Time to forget COVID and other worries for a while.

The day began in Westminster Abbey. Great people from all countries with many traditions came together. The servant King was annointed to the accompaniment of wonderful music including an anthem written by Gambier Parry who once lived at Highnam Count in Gloucester.

Two days later in Gloucester Cathedral, Princess Anne, sister of King Charles visited Gloucester Cathedral to attend another service of celebrations. As in Westminster Abbey the walls echoed as the choir sang. It was a happy, positive, occasion. The Bishop leading the service was a caring lady named Rachael.

Turn back in time to the year 1216, we are still in Gloucester. This was the year when a young boy of ten years old, was told he would be crowned King of England. Henry was taken from his home in Kingsholm, accompanied by his Mother Isabella of

Angouleme to the Cathedral. They had been living in Kingsholm as a safe place away from Henry's father King John.

In a mysterious way John had died leaving many questions unanswered and an immediate problem to be solved. The King of France was in Calais hoping to claim the English throne. Little Henry needed to be crowned without delay. All was quickly arranged. Henry was crowned in Gloucester Cathedral. His father had carelessly lost his crown whilst crossing a river, so his Mother's bracelet was used instead. There was certainly a lot of excitement on that day as people of Gloucester arrived in great numbers, and cheered the Young King Henry III Gloucester was a happy place that day.

Now back again to 2023 but still in Gloucester Cathedral. We find another young boy of ten years.

This time his name is James he too has just

left his home to celebrate the crowning of a new King of England. He too has a part to play, not as a King but as a chorister in the wonderful choir raising the roof to welcome Princess Anne. After the joyous occasion, James presented Anne with a posy of flowers in the cloisters. 1216 or 2023, Two young boys took their place in the history of Gloucester.

Long live the King!

We need the knowledge of the past to manage th present and to plan for the futures.

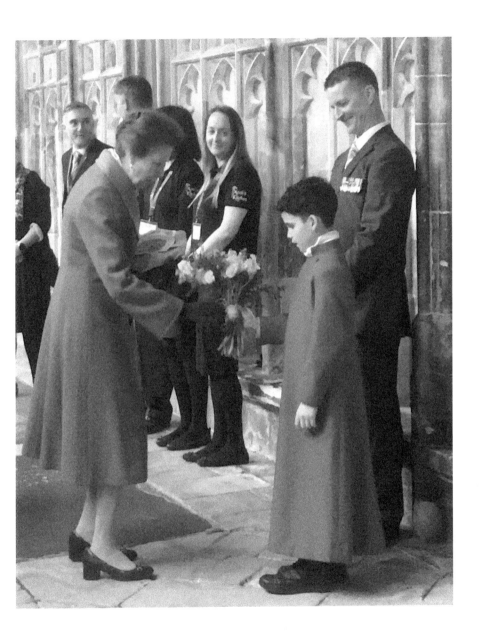

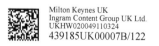
Milton Keynes UK
Ingram Content Group UK Ltd.
UKHW020049110324
439185UK00007B/122